Lecture Reprint Number 5

A Health Pattern To Live By

by Bernard Jensen, Ph.D., D.C., N.D.

Revised and edited by Jon D. Jensen

Acknowledgements

I acknowledge and give thanks to Betty Norlin for being such a wonderful friend, my editor and for continually encouraging me and assisting me on my book writing/editing journey. Author of *"Our Bodies: The Optimal Design."*

www.bettynorlin.com   www.whatisholistichealth.com

I acknowledge and give thanks to Daylin Anderson for help with editing and typing with this lecture reprint booklet series.

I acknowledge and give thanks to Gary and Jeanne Nichols. They have given their expertise in editing and marketing as well as assisting me with my grandfather's videos taking them from video to DVD. They have always supported me whether it was creating an office space, assistance with writing, promoting me or help with giving lectures. Thank you both!

Copyright

Copyright © 2021 by Jon D. Jensen

Because of the dynamic nature of the Internet, any web addresses or links contained in this book may have changed since publication and may no longer be valid.

Paperback

ISBN-9781688464971

Disclaimer

Any information given in this book is not intended to be taken as a replacement for medical advice. Any person with a condition requiring medical attention should consult a qualified health professional.

Introduction

My name is Jon Jensen and I have been involved in the holistic health field for many years. I published a nutrition book, "A Simple Guide to Healthy Living" as a way to communicate with people outside my client base about information I feel is key to a healthy life. It is available on Amazon and my website at www.jensenholistichealth.com.

I've had the idea to republish these health booklets for many years. My intention for editing, revising and publishing my grandfather's 21 lecture reprint booklets is rooted in my desire to continue his legacy of teaching right living through health and nutrition. Dr. Bernard Jensen spent his lifetime helping others to achieve health through education and his writing, and I feel strongly that the message is needed now more than ever.

I've always marveled how one person could write so many books and still travel, receive numerous awards, teach classes on Iridology, rejuvenation, regeneration and tissue cleansing. He recorded his lectures onto cassette tapes and eventually had a series of videos that corresponded with many of his books. These lecture reprints are the product of his first lectures, typed up and stapled into booklets and originally sold for ninety-nine cents each. This started a pattern where he would write and self-publish many books over his lifetime.

Bernard Jensen, Ph.D., D.C., N.D.

One of the greatest healers the world has ever known. Dr. Bernard Jensen spent over 60 years as a pioneer in the holistic health field, helping to pave the way for the alternative health revolution that we are now experiencing.

Dr. Jensen began his career at the West Coast Chiropractic College where he became the youngest Chiropractor in the state of California. He traveled extensively in search of health knowledge, a search that led him to over 65 countries to observe the lifestyles of the people and their various ways of eating. Each place provided a different health secret.

Throughout his career, Dr. Jensen wrote and published over 60 books, a quarterly magazine for several years, a cassette and video tape series and a slide presentation for his Iridology class. After working with over 350,000 patients, Dr. Jensen firmly believed that nutrition is the greatest single therapy to be applied in the holistic healing arts and that, "We must treat the patient, not just the disease."

Born on March 25, 1908, to parents of Danish descent, Eugen and Anna Jensen, Jorgen Bernard Jensen was raised in Stockton, California, then a small rural town in one of the richest agricultural valleys of the state. The unexpected death of his mother at age 29 from tuberculosis and consumption left the three children to be raised by their father, Eugen Jensen who was a chiropractor. Very little has been written about Bernard's early life growing up in Stockton or his brother and sister. There are a few comments in lectures he made about his father, who was very strict and analytical.

Early in life, young Bernard displayed the qualities needed for his future work. His penchant for being critical as well as a serious perfectionist blended with his sensitive, competitive, spiritual-minded personality to arm him with an unusual perspective that opened the doors to the unconventional life he was soon to enter. But before that path was firmly set, several intense learning experiences occurred which determined the direction he was to take.

Being his own worst obstacle, restless and never satisfied, he would rather study and read a book than eat or sleep. His father was a chiropractor, and young Bernard followed in his path. When he was 18 years old, Bernard entered the West Coast Chiropractic College in Oakland, California. During his years of study, Bernard burned the midnight oil while holding down as many as two outside jobs simultaneously. The strain was immense. The capacity to push forward and the ability to persevere doggedly toward a goal were firmly established, but there was a price to pay. Bernard supported himself by working at a dairy in his spare time, and the long hours of work and study, along with poor food habits, took a heavy toll on Bernard's health. After receiving his diploma in 1929, Dr. Bernard Jensen went into practice, opening his first office in Oakland, California. He focused intently on the task of his calling which was to offer a helping hand to those suffering and in need. Dr. Bernard Jensen's devotion was complete, the hours long, his personal needs forgotten. By this time, the sacrificing of many years began to demand attention. His health began to fail. A Medical Doctor diagnosed his condition as bronchiectasis, an often-fatal lung condition, with no known cure at the time. "There is nothing I can do for you," he was told. The young man refused to give up, searching out a Seventh Day Adventist Medical Doctor who taught him basic nutritional principles, told Dr. Bernard Jensen to leave junk food alone and promptly presented him with a maintenance program involving natural health that emphasized the return to a pure, natural and whole foods regimen. Following this program brought excellent results. Dr. Bernard Jensen was soon on the way back to health and renewed vitality. A great turning point had occurred. To be able to study nutrition and discover the laws of right living became his burning desire. Dr. Bernard Jensen turned the experience of what he learned from the Seventh Day Adventist Medical Doctor about the holistic approach into helping his patients get better and teach them how to prevent themselves from getting sick. Dr. Bernard Jensen began taking breathing exercises with Thomas Gaines, once an instructor for the New York City Police Department. Slowly, his health returned, and his lungs eventually healed completely.

Using this knowledge in working with his patients the results were dramatic and effective. Dr. Bernard Jensen's attention was now riveted in this direction. Natural therapeutics became his healing mode, setting the pattern for the rest of his life. He began to travel in search of more knowledge and information.

Dr. Bernard Jensen opened his first office in Oakland, California, in 1929. He later moved to Los Angeles and expanded his practice to include branch offices at Long Beach and Santa Monica, with several chiropractors working under him. Such success had not come about overnight. In Chicago, Dr. Bernard Jensen took his post-graduate work at the National Chiropractic College and later from the Los Angeles Chiropractic College closer to home. Upon returning to California, he began an intensive study and investigation of something he was recently just learning about, the subject of iridology.

Dr. Bernard Jensen used Rocine's work as the basis for the programs used in his sanitariums. First, a 25-bed sanitarium in San Leandro, California, then others in Ben Lomond and Alta Dena, and finally an 85-bed sanitarium at hidden Valley Health Ranch in Escondido, California. The sanitariums were quite successful, demonstrating the effectiveness of Rocine's ideas in working with patients. It was the Hidden Valley Health Ranch in Escondido that provided the greatest opportunity for applying the rules of right living. People in search of health and rejuvenation came to the ranch from all over the world to learn the principles that Dr. Bernard Jensen believed in, practiced, and taught.

Proper nutrition, together with sunshine, rest, exercise, fresh air and positive attitudes helped thousands of patients at Dr. Bernard Jensen's Sanitariums leave behind the symptoms of chronic diseases that they have developed. After working with several hundred thousand patients, Dr. Bernard Jensen concluded that nutrition is the single most important therapy to be used in the healing arts.

Patients came from all over the world, some to stay at his sanitariums, others for outpatient consultations and still others to attend his classes in rejuvenation and Food Studies. Thousands of New Zealanders formed clubs to follow his dietetic advice, filling out the over 350,000 people he reached, accumulated over the years. He acquired a multitude of experiences from these people individually and in group studies, acquiring information and summing it up for use in his healing work and writing.

Dr. Bernard Jensen visited the Hunza Valley, where disease, doctors, dentist and hospitals were practically nonexistent and where there were no jails, prisons or police, because there was no crime. One of Dr. Bernard Jensen's highlights of that trip was staying as a guest of the Mir of Hunza's palace for 10 days.

Dr. Bernard Jensen visited the Caucasus Mountains in the USSR to meet a 153-year-old man who had stopped riding horseback a few years earlier only because of his doctor's orders. Dr. Bernard Jensen traveled to Vilcabamba, Ecuador, where heart patients were able to recuperate so marvelously. Everywhere Dr. Bernard Jensen went, he brought back some new remedy or approach to integrate into the system he taught his patients.

Dr. Bernard Jensen received his Ph.D. at the age of 75 from the University of Humanistic Studies, San Diego, California.

Dr. Bernard Jensen retired from active chiropractic practice in 1978, and devoted himself to teaching, writing and lecturing on the subjects of nutrition, rejuvenation and iridology. Around this time, Dr. Bernard Jensen completed work on a two-hour feature film titled, *"World Search for Health, Happiness and Long Life,"* narrated by actor Dennis Weaver.

The Academy of Science in Paris awarded Dr.

Bernard Jensen a medal in 1971 for exceptional services rendered to humanity. Also, in the same year, 1971, Dr. Bernard Jensen received an honorary doctorate from the Center for the Study of Human Sciences in Lisbon, Portugal.

At a ceremony in San Remo, Italy in 1973, Dr. Bernard Jensen was presented the Ignatz Von Peczely International Iridology Gold Medal by the World Congress of Scientific Medicine, an organization embracing many medical and health disciplines.

A congress of health professionals at Aix-en Provence, France, in 1974, recognized Dr. Bernard Jensen with an award for his "valuable contribution in the field of iridology."

Then in 1975, the International Naturopathic Association honored Dr. Bernard Jensen for his service to mankind through his work in the fields of health, Iridology, and nutrition.

Knighted into the Order of St. John of Malta in 1978 for his humanitarian work in the field of health, Dr. Bernard Jensen was awarded the cross of St. John at a special ceremony in New York City. This Order is the oldest chivalric organization in the world, tracing its origin back to the time preceding the first Crusade.

In 1981, at the Fifth Annual Herb Symposium, the Agnes Arber Distinguished Service award was presented to Dr. Bernard Jensen for his contributions to the current "herb renaissance."

In 1982, the National Health Federation honored Dr.

Bernard Jensen with its Pioneer Doctor of the Year award at its annual convention in Long Beach, California.

In 1982, Dr. Bernard Jensen traveled to Brussels, Belgium to accept the 1982 Dag Hammarskjold award of the Pax Mundi Academy, an international organization which presents annual awards to those in the arts and sciences who have made outstanding contributions in their fields. The award, in the category of scientific merit, was for "the exceptional services rendered to collective humanity… toward international cooperation and solidarity…" Dr. Bernard Jensen was personally congratulated on his award by U. S. Ambassador, Charles Price.

In 1988 Dr. Bernard Jensen held his 80th Birthday Celebration at the Town and Country Hotel in San Diego, California, where people came from all over the world to celebrate his 80 years of life and work in the holistic health field.

In 1993 he was presented with a PhD. in natural healing arts and sciences from Westbrook University, where his iridology course was part of the school curriculum.

In 1995 Dr. Bernard Jensen's grandson Jon stayed by his grandfather's side after Dr. Jensen became paralyzed from the waist down from a car accident. Jon was right there every day of his grandfather's plan to walk again. With a big sign on the wall in front of Dr. Jensen's bed where he could see it every day that said, "LUCKY BOY." Every day consisted of many different healing modalities and supplements. Jon would travel to the Hidden Valley Health Ranch in the early morning and watch while Apolinar, Dr. Jensen's main ranch worker, milked the goat for

Dr. Jensen's fresh morning goat milk drink. After breakfast and supplements, there was stretching, going to the gym and massages 2 times a week. A physical therapist came in every day to assist in the gym and to stretch the muscles.

Jon would drive his grandfather and grandmother Marie to Los Angeles twice a week for chiropractic adjustments and frequency therapy, treating the whole body, mind, and spirit, and being involved in every aspect of what the doctors called a **"Miracle"—as his grandfather walked again on his own.** Jon is writing more on the entire recovery process and will publish it through Amazon.

In 1998 and 1999 Dr. Bernard Jensen received awards from the IIPA for his work in iridology.

On February 22, 2001 a month before his 93rd birthday, Dr. Bernard Jensen passed away at 92 years old.

The short biography above about Dr. Bernard Jensen is a small part of a larger biography I am writing about my grandfather's life. If you are interested in learning more I will be blogging and have more information at www.bernardjensen.org.

In the 21 lecture reprint booklets you'll see products or foods that might not be commonly found today. I left some things in to give the flavor of that time period and what he was thinking at that time. I also left in quotes or sayings from that era. I edited misspellings and grammatical errors. But overall, I feel that these booklets give down to earth advice and can still be regarded as basic knowledge in the mainstream health field today. A lot of his products are no longer available, but you can find what remains on my website, www.jensenholistichealth.com.

I hope you enjoy these lecture reprint booklets as much as I do and take them for what they are; a novelty and glimpse of the past. A simple approach of one of the early promoters of healthy living. Alongside such greats of that era like Paul Bragg, Jack LaLanne, Dr. Max Gerson, V.E. Irons and Dr. Bronner at the beginning of a health revolution.

Jon D. Jensen, CMH

HEALTH PATTERN TO LIVE BY

"My purpose is to serve and I must serve my purpose."

Bernard Jensen, Ph.D., D.C, N.D.

For quite some time I have been searching for a means of bringing, not to just the few that I can work with at the sanitarium, but to everyone who wants it, a program which would enable the individual to establish and maintain himself in an enlightened, spiritual consciousness, with a healthy mind that could be expressed through the channels provided for by a healthy physical body.

I have learned much from my patients at the sanitarium. They have been my guinea pigs, my proving ground. They have helped me to give this program to you.

I am tempted to talk only about spiritual, theoretical things, about my dreams, but I have found that we have to tie the physical and the mental world, the whole of our life together. A "program of living," includes the whole body.

While I was in Europe, I kept notes on some topics I want to discuss with you. They have there what is called the Kure Haus (Cure House) where they use water treatments, Kneipp baths, for health regeneration.

I want to develop such a cure plan. When I talk about a *cure*, you understand that I do not mean I cure you. I cannot cure you as you must cure yourselves, but I can help you cease setting up causes that produce ill effects and start setting up causes that produce good and healthful effects.

You can break old habits that destroy you physically and demoralize you mentally. You can set up new habits that will make you vitally alive physically, mentally and spiritually.

We have to find a health premise in what we do. I want to work out a simple system that you can follow to keep in good health. It will be well rounded out, simple and fundamental, a program that will include ways to think, ways to deal with life and how to cope with your environment. It will deal with ways to meet physical, mental and spiritual needs.

There are certain health axioms that are undeniable. For instance: "A serene mind supersedes a relaxed body." This truth is so fundamental that you cannot get away from it. If you want the mind at ease, the spirit must be at ease. If you want the body at ease, you have to have the mind at ease. So, ease of mind begets ease of body; that is a law. This law is so definite and so fundamental, that unless you realize it, you would never know what it is to be in good health.

You must live on natural foods and that too is a law. Water is a food, but most important of all, do not forget that BREATH is a FOOD. You can go without water and other foods for long periods, but the supply of air is quickly dissipated in the body and must be renewed within a matter of minutes to sustain LIFE.

Joy is necessary for good health. It is a law. You cannot feel blue and feel well. If you are going to have the blues all the time, you are going to have a bad liver and indigestion. If you have indigestion, you can have anything from that time on because indigestion is the beginning of every disease.

So put your mind in order, at ease. Chaotic, confused thinking is diseased thinking. Try exercising your will power over your thoughts for just five minutes. You will find it is very difficult to make your thoughts follow a straight line. Stray thoughts will keep creeping in, deflecting you from your goal of straight thinking.

When you are thinking right you create a magnetic field of thought about you which will cause others, who are thinking along the same lines, to gravitate to you. And "where two or three are gathered together in MY NAME, there also am I." In this agreement, this "union of thought," there is a bond which is hard to break. And when we have achieved this "straight thinking," this "union of thought," we are ready to tune in intuitionally to the source of all knowledge and receive, and in return, give.

You are unable to do this if you continue to indulge in chaotic, disjointed, loose thinking; hateful, vengeful or fearful thinking. That is like static on a radio. When you have static, you have nothing but a lot of "sound in confusion and fury." You cannot possibly receive a "message" or catch the music of Nature or the rhythm of natural life, you know this is true, you know that "static" is not right. You must tune in with that which is constructive, in order that the forces of right may be strengthened by this agreement of right thinking in unison.

It is also a law, that if you do not use your body you will lose it. Keep your body limber and your mind flexible by using them. If you have a "fixation" in the mind it can cause a fixation in the body. That means that a fixed fear, or hatred in the mind, can turn up as a fixation in the body in the form of arthritis, bad posture, or may result in favoring one part of the body more than the other. If these fixations of the body are the result of fixations in the mind, then we have to open up new channels in the mind. When you relax and let go of these tensions in the mind, then the tension in the muscles let go.

Through faith and relaxation many spiritual healings take place because through "faith," which is "unconscious straight intelligence," people relax and let go of their fixations and tensions which have crippled them. I have seen a spine come right out from under a shoulder blade in just one treatment, when a man just put his hand there. The person believed, relaxed, let go in God and the dis-ease disappeared.

Many of us hold on to a pattern of living that is difficult for the body to follow. If it is not a good pattern, it is a disease pattern. Develop a healthy pattern to live by.

I believe one of the greatest crimes of today is the fact that 97% of all money spent with doctors is spent for cures, trying to get well after you are sick. Less than 3% of all money spent on doctors and doctoring in the health field is spent in the prevention of disease.

In other words, less than 3% of billions of dollars is spent on eliminating the *cause*, while 97% is spent in attempting to *cure* the effects. The sensible thing to do would be to eliminate the cause of disease. Always trying to "treat" disease is like constantly bailing water out of a leaky boat, instead of mending the boat.

We would not need vitamins and mineral tablets and we would not be doctor chasers, doctor shoppers, if we lived even half-way healthfully.

I do not like to call the routine I am giving you a "cure day" routine. Perhaps instead of developing a cure day program, we should try to make every day of our life a day of "pure living." We would then have no ills that necessitate a cure day. A good motto might be, "Make your day a pure day and you will never need a cure day."

In this pure day routine, we should consider establishing habits that keep us well. We should learn to eat pure, natural foods, breathe pure air and think pure thoughts. We may not be able to do this all at once, but gradually, as we use our will power to establish good habits, we will find it is easier to maintain habits that give us freedom than it is to maintain habits which cripple our bodies, frustrate our minds and leave us spiritually floundering.

Combing your hair is a habit that may not particularly help your health any. But it helps you get along with people; to attract the best in other people by expressing yourself with a good front. How about your stomach, your teeth, your liver? Are they also being cared for, so that you can express yourself to the fullest in your living?

The average doctor dies at the age of 49! The average person lives until 59 or 60. We find that the greatest knowledge or wisdom is given to the world by men of older years. We can only give the "wise things," when we have a good body and an alert mind with which to gather in and to give out. So, why should we be crawling during what should be the wisest days of our life? We should be able to walk, to give, to have bodies that can do the things we want to do, in order to be 100% successful in our work. When I speak of being successful, I do not mean, especially, successful in making money.

If it is making money we desire more than anything else, then let us learn to use it for good. The person who is worried about money and is after only material things in life has fears regarding his health and the new day; is afraid he cannot carry on. He has developed an inward fear; his faith is in reverse. He does not have faith in the finer things of life. He has faith only in material things; thus, he has a poor pattern to live by. If this man changed his pattern, he would find joy in living, rather than misery.

Many people are actually "enjoying poor health." They enjoy going to the doctor, enjoy talking about their operations. Their thinking is all wrong!

The time is coming when people will deride you if you say you have diabetes. They will tell you have been drinking soda pop, eating too many refined starches, too much white sugar and candy. If you say you have arthritis, they will say, "You've been having too much ice cream, too many pickles, and too many acid-forming foods." If you have high blood pressure, people will say, "It serves you right, you have been drinking too much coffee and eating too many doughnuts."

Doctors are not privileged to be well, any more than their patients. The average doctor is just like the patient, he does not have time for health. There are so many other things they think are more important. A doctor is bound by a feeling of duty where his patient is concerned, patients cannot be "put off until tomorrow." We are all going at this business backwards. Why wait until people have spent 20 30 years breaking themselves down? Doctors should teach people to live correctly; then make sure that they live correctly. If they do not, then Nature has demands which she makes upon them.

I believe that I am in the best work possible. That is EDUCATING people to live correctly rather than to treat people. Suppressive treatments only move bad habits around, move a pain from the head to the stomach, from one diseased part of the body to another, from an acute condition to a sub-acute condition, from a sub-acute condition to a chronic one. This type of treatment only assuages the discomfort of dis-ease.

You may have a share in health but in order to have it, you are going to have to live in such a way that you are able to claim it. Health, like everything else, is something you must earn.

I am being honest with you when I tell you that you cannot get well because of what I say or do for you. You must cooperate. I cannot pour health into you and you do not have enough money to buy health. You cannot secure it from me, even though I have practiced for twenty years, and I am supposed to know something. I say again, it is you who must do something about your health. If you do not take yourself in hand, there is no hope for you. If you just sit on the sofa and do nothing about it, you are going to remain on that sofa. No one can carry anyone else. All I can do, all any doctor can do, is to inspire you to a better way to live.

You have heard that old saying about how "the doctor was a success, the operation was a success, but the patient died." We do not have failures if we look at them the right way. Many people come into our office to be built up for operations, but after they are built up, they do not need the operations.

On the following pages, I am outlining a routine for you and also telling you about the foods that are not good for you. I know that many of you will say, after you have followed this routine for a week, "I've done this now for a whole week and nothing is happening." You try this routine for three months and then tell me whether "anything is happening," or not!

Anyone who follows this routine for three months will never go back to bad habits of living.

Let us take a searching look at what causes depleted body tissues, tissues that have lost their elasticity and tone, jittery nerves and upset glandular condition.

The body, like a furnace, requires fuel and oxygen to create combustion to furnish heat or energy. If you put slack coal into your furnace and keep all the dampers closed, you get very little heat and the furnace becomes filled with clinkers. The same is true of your body. If you fill it with devitalized foods and your breathing is shallow, your whole system becomes clogged with waste materials, and eventually the fire goes out within you. In other words, you will lack energy; the tissues, nerves and glands will become dis-eased and finally you give up the struggle, your nerve energy being depleted, and your tissues having reached the extreme "acid point."

There are many reasons why the foods that most people eat today are lacking in nutritional value. The first mistake we make is in buying foods that have been "refined." White flour and white sugar have been so thoroughly bleached and depleted of all vitality and life-giving force, that the government has compelled commercial users and distributors to replace some of the vitamins and minerals, artificially. Unfortunately, this replacement is of inorganic vitamins and minerals, which the body does not assimilate.

We see bread advertised that is supposed to build bodies eight different ways and this advertised bread is white bread. There is only one way we know of to build a healthy body and that is by a well-balanced diet of natural foods, prepared in the health way, which we teach in our lectures and books.

Most people judge food by its color. Harmful preservatives such as coal tar and baking soda have been added indiscriminately to preserve the color of foods. These preservatives may keep the food from spoiling over a longer period of time and heighten the color, but they do not preserve the minerals and vitamins in foods. In addition to destroying the minerals and vitamins in the foods which it "preserves," coal tar becomes an irritant in the body.

Spices, which are also irritating, are used copiously in the preservation of foods. If you are one of those persons who "relishes" your condiments, you will sooner or later find yourself in a "pickle" and when they "catsup" with you will have fifty-seven varieties of twinges, aches, groans and miseries. Do you realize that 60% of the food today is canned with white sugar or has white sugar in it? It is hard to believe that an average of 116 lbs. of white sugar is being eaten by each person every year. Someone is eating more than that for we are not eating any in our home.

Food today is being grown on soil that is "worn out;" soil that lacks the minerals and vitamins which the plant itself must have to become a healthy plant, capable of passing on to us and to animals a rich content of minerals and vitamins. Farmers must be educated on the replenishment of soil so it will grow plants that bring to us the proper vitamins and minerals in our foods. Milk and milk products are deficient in vitamins and minerals if cows are fed devitalized food.

The next blunder is in the preparation of food. We boil it in open utensils and the kitchen walls and ceiling get the benefit of the vitamins that go up in the steam. Or we fry it using excessive heat, which destroys the vitamin value. In this new day of jet propulsion and atomic energy, many of you are still using grandma's old black skillet that she brought across the plains in a covered wagon. If you must keep it for its sentimental value, hang it on the wall and leave it there. Or better yet, you might plant an organic garden in it and decorate the kitchen windowsill. Many of you are using cooking utensils made of harmful metals and they corrode and contaminate the food that is cooked in them.

The average person has a minimum of one ton of food passing through his body each year. How much of it is "foodless" food? We are not spending our money wisely, not eating wisely.

Natural Foods for a Correct Diet

The body is made up of certain elements. Replacement of these elements are necessary as cells wear out and are replaced by new cells. If the foods we eat are deficient in these elements, the new cells will be deficient and consequently will be unhealthy. Your body must have calcium, silicon, iodine, magnesium, manganese, zinc, and trace elements that many chemists do not even know about. The best way to obtain these elements is from natural foods.

Make a habit of applying the following general diet regime to your everyday living. THIS IS A HEALTHFUL WAY TO LIVE BECAUSE, when followed, you do not have to think of vitamins, mineral elements or calories. You may, however, have to have specific instructions for any specific troubles you may have already developed, but first, make this daily regime automatic.

The best diet for each day is two different fruits, at least four to six vegetables, one protein and one starch, with fruit or vegetable juices between meals. Eat at least two green leafy vegetables a day. Consider this regime a dietetic law.

BEFORE BREAKFAST

Upon arising, take any natural unsweetened fruit juice, such as grapefruit, grape, pineapple or orange juice. This is to be taken one-half before breakfast. Prune, fig, apple and black cherry juices are exceptionally good. Between fruit juice and breakfast follow this program:

Skin Brushing:

When the skin is covered with clothes the dead epidermis is not thrown off as it would be if no clothes were worn. Clothes do not allow a complete evaporation of the toxic material in the body that should come through the skin and be thrown off. So, when we wear clothes this toxic elimination must be brushed away. All eliminative organs should be taken care of and the elimination that takes place through the skin is just as important as any other elimination.

Brushing the skin is done by using a flesh massage brush. The brush should be used dry before the bath, not in the bath. The skin has to eliminate two to four pounds of toxic waste per day and this is the same kind of toxic waste material that is eliminated through the bowels, kidneys and lungs. It is important to allow this elimination to take place through the skin. Skin rashes are caused by faulty skin elimination. Skin rashes may be avoided by skin brushing, plus proper elimination through the bowels, kidneys and lungs.

Exercising:

Hiking, deep breathing or playing.

Shower:

Start warm and cool off until your breath quickens. Never shower immediately upon rising.

BREAKFAST

STEWED FRUIT, ONE STARCH AND HEALTH DRINK
 . . . (See starches and health drinks listed under "lunch").

or

TWO FRUITS, ONE PROTEIN AND HEALTH DRINK FRUITS: any kind such as, unsulphured apricots, prunes, figs, (soak dried fruits) melon, grapes, peaches, pears, berries, or baked apple, which may be sprinkled with some ground nuts, or dripped with nut butter. If time of year suggests any other fruit, use it.

SUGGESTIONS: Sliced figs and cream; half cantaloupe with strawberries. Any TWO FRUITS with creamed cottage cheese and honey, if you are a heavy worker and you feel as though fruit is not enough for you. Almond butter, or cashew nut butter are quite nourishing and can be used on fruits. Eat an egg with fruit and vary these from day to day. Also, yogurt mixed with fruit, one or two different fruits like berries and apricots, topped with wheat germ and rice polishing. If you want to sweeten this a little bit, you could use a little apple concentrate or a little honey. This makes a very good breakfast.

10:30 A.M. VEGETABLE BROTH

Vital Broth—Excellent for Elimination

2 cups carrot tops

3 cups celery stalk

1/2 Tsp. Savita

2 cups celery tops

2 Qts. distilled water

2 cups potato peeling (cut 1/2 inch thick)

Add a carrot or onion for flavor if desired.

Finely chop or grate vegetables. Bring slowly to a boil, simmer approximately twenty minutes. Just use broth after straining. Note: *(c) following a fruit means that it is a citrus fruit.

LUNCH

(For Mid-day or Evening)

RAW SALAD, ONE STARCH, as listed, and HEALTH DRINK—with rye crisp, cornbread or bran muffins. Get salad suggestions from Dr. Jensen's LIVE FOODS AND TOTAL HEALTH book.

RAW SALAD

VEGETABLES

Tomatoes (c)

Lettuce Romaine

Endive

Celery

Grated Carrots

Onions

Cabbage (s)

Peppers

Radishes

Avocado

Parsley

Watercress

Any raw "salad vegetable"

STARCH

Barley (natural—unpeeled)

Baked Potato

Baked Banana (or at least dead ripe)

Steamed brown rice or wild rice

Yellow corn meal

Bread (whole wheat, rye, or soybean)

Sandwiches (use above breads)

Cereals (Dr. Jackson meal, syldex,

Roman meal, shredded wheat and

other whole grain products)

Note: *(c) means citrus. (s) sulphur foods.

DRINKS: Vegetable broth, coffee substitute, buttermilk, raw milk, oat straw tea, alfalfa mint tea, or any health drink.

3:00 O'CLOCK

FRUIT OF ANY KIND, such as: dates, apples, figs, peaches, etc. Fruit juices or vegetable juices.

DINNER

(for Mid-day or Evening)

Dinner should consist of a SMALL RAW SALAD, TWO COOKED VEGETABLES, ONE PROTEIN, AND A BROTH or HEALTH DRINK if desired.

COOKED VEGETABLES

Peas

String Beans

Artichokes

Carrots

Beets

Turnips

Spinach

Beet Tops

Cauliflower (s)

Zucchini

Sprouts (s)

Swiss Chard

Egg Plant

Cabbage (s)

Onions (s)

Mustard Greens (s)

Summer Squash

Or any vegetable other than potatoes.

ONE PROTEIN

ONCE A WEEK: FISH. Use white fish with fins and scales, such as sole, halibut, trout or sea trout. If complete vegetarian, use soybeans, lima beans, cottage cheese, etc. Other good meat substitutes are canned baby soybeans, almond butter. THREE TIMES A WEEK: MEAT. Use only lean meat. Never use pork or fats. If complete vegetarian use soybeans, lima beans, cottage cheese, eggs and hard curd cheeses. TWICE A WEEK: COTTAGE CHEESE.

Drinks:

Broth or Health Beverages. If you have a protein with this dinner meal, a health dessert is allowed, but not recommended. (See suggestions in Live Foods and Total Health cookbook.)

Never eat protein and starch together. (Notice how they are separated.)

You may exchange your noon meal for your evening meal but follow the same regime. It takes exercise to handle raw food and we generally get more after our noon meal. That is why the big raw salad is advised at noon. Starches are also best eaten at noon, as they are energy foods; so if one eats sandwiches, it should be at noon.

Fruit salads may be substituted for any of these meals. (See **LIVE FOODS AND TOTAL HEALTH** for suggested fruit salads). If you do not feel hungry or any too well, a fruit salad is the best food to eat.

BEFORE RETIRING, go through your slanting board exercises.

SLANTING BOARD EXERCISES

Use ankle straps while doing these exercises. Raise foot end of board 18 inches from floor.

Lie full length, with head down, allowing gravity to help the abdominal organs into their proper position. For best results lie on board at least one half hour.

1. Stretch the abdomen by putting arms above head for about five minutes. Relax about five minutes and repeat.

2. Pull up abdominal organs while holding breath. Exhale, relax and repeat. Move the organs back and forth by drawing them upward, then allowing them to go back to a relaxed position. Do these rhythmically ten or fifteen times. Relax completely and repeat.

3. Pat abdomen vigorously with cupped hands. Lean to one side, then to the other, patting the stretched side.

Remove feet from straps and hold on to handles while doing the following exercises:

4. Bend knees and legs at hips. While in this relaxed position (a) turn head from side to side five or six times; (b) lift the head slightly and rotate in circles three or four times.

5. Lift legs to a vertical position and rotate outward in circles eight or ten times.

6. Grasp the edge of the board and raise your legs straight up. Inhale and lower your legs to the board. Exhale, as you pull your legs up again. Do these four or five times. Rest and relax. Repeat about twelve times if *not fatigued.*

Relax and rest, completely letting the blood circulate in the head for a while.

How to Make a Slanting Exercise Board

The board should be eighteen to twenty inches wide; made of five-plywood, three-fourths inch thick. Side handles are made by cutting a slit hole three-quarters of an inch in from the edge of the board, twenty-four inches down from the head end of the board. A strap fastened near the foot end holds ankles to keep the body from sliding and to bring the body to a sitting position when exercising.

If you prefer to purchase a slanting board instead of making one yourself, write to Doctor Jensen for name of manufacturer.

RULES OF EATING

1. If not entirely comfortable in mind and body from the previous mealtime, you should miss the next meal.

2. Do not eat unless you have a keen desire for the plainest food.

3. Do not eat beyond your needs.

4. Be sure to thoroughly masticate your food.

5. Miss meals if in pain, emotionally upset, not hungry, chilled, overheated and during acute illness.

If we are to follow such a food regime as the above successfully, we must know where and how to obtain these foods. The best place to obtain most of them is in your health food stores.

What do we mean by natural foods? Natural foods are whole grain foods that have been grown in good soil, rich in the mineral elements that the plant needs to be a healthy plant. They have not been polished, for polishing robs the grains of much of their rich mineral value. Good vegetables are rich in their natural colors, crisp and firm, denoting that they have been grown in soil organically complete with all minerals. Raw milk, that has not been pasteurized or sterilized or heated or treated in any way, and that has been obtained from well cared for goats or cows, that have been properly fed and inspected, would be considered as a good *natural* food. Milk must be carefully handled at all times to keep it clean.

It has been proven, when plants are grown in organically rich soil, that an infected plant, placed alongside of a healthy plant, cannot affect or infect the healthy plant. The same is true of animals and human beings. They are capable of withstanding diseases when they are healthy. These same principles hold true concerning the growing of nuts and fruits.

It will be a waste of your time, however, to buy food that is perfect and then not eat a balanced diet, or if you do not properly prepare your food.

AIR AS FOOD

AIR is the most vitally important food of all, as you cannot live but a matter of minutes without it. Fresh, clean air supplies us with oxygen and also with nitrogen.

Breathing Correctly

The average person does not breathe correctly. Here is an exercise which will do a lot of good. It is what we call "sniff breathing" or "confidence breath." When out walking divide your steps into sevens. During the first three steps, "sniff in" three times, inhaling without exhaling at all. The last "sniff in" really fills the lungs completely. On the fourth step, let all air out with a quick exhalation. During steps five, six and seven, make no effort toward breathing. Then start over again, as before, breathing while walking. This will help to clean the catarrh out of the nose, lungs and bronchial structure. It is very important to do this at the beginning of the day, so that your oxygen intake will remain at a maximum during the day. "Sniff" breathing develops the lung structure, so that when you are relaxed your lungs are at full capacity. Sniff breathing also develops the distance between the ribs; makes the cartilage between the ribs more limber, pliable, and active, so that breathing is an easier job on the body.

COOKING OF FOODS

USE STAINLESS STEEL UTENSILS THAT DO NOT BECOME ERODED and that have lids: that are made to do waterless cooking, as there is enough moisture in all fruits and vegetables to cook them. If water is added, there is a loss of vitamins and minerals into the water. By using cooking utensils that are covered, you do not lose vitamins and minerals in the steam.

Use moderate heat in cooking, as excessive heat destroys vitamins.

Sunshine, Exercise and Relaxation:

We are not children of the sun, as we used to be. We have not developed a pigment in our skin that enables it to withstand a great deal of sunshine, so we can overdo sunbathing. Ten minutes a day is all that is necessary, but do not go over fifteen or twenty minutes. Especially, get the sunshine on the long bones of the body and the back. In ten or fifteen minutes of sunshine a day, you can build into the body all the vitamin D that is necessary to last the body for three days.

The habit of going to the beach once a week and burning yourselves "to a crisp," is a devitalizing and definitely not a building process. There are a great many skin diseases developing today, because of an excessive amount of sunshine.

Many bodies have been filled with coal tar products, with drugs and with such chemicals as sulphur, for instance. When you go through a sunbathing and diet program, you start a process of elimination of all matters foreign and unfavorable to the body; this elimination works through the skin, as well as through the other organs of elimination.

Everyone should learn to play and it is absolutely imperative that you learn to relax. At any one time, do not exercise more than three or four minutes and then rest. The exercises do no good without rest. In fact, the relaxation you get from exercising and then resting is the only good you get out of it. Without relaxation we bum our bodies up in a few years; whereas, we could live many, many more years by knowing how to relax.

Swimming is one of the best physical exercises and it is at the same time a pleasure. Lying prone in the water, and pulling the arms forward and then backward, pulls the organs toward the shoulders, and this action of swimming allows the water to massage the entire body. I believe swimming will do more for you than anything else, from an exercise standpoint.

Going Barefoot

Our civilized life requires everyone to wear shoes, but we should go barefoot as often as possible. Walk on the grass, preferably when the morning dew is still upon it, or at least, walk barefoot outside, for at least five minutes a day; sand walking is also very good.

No one who wears shoes can use his feet properly and so it is very necessary to walk barefoot at least five minutes a day—no less. When you move your fingers, note how you move muscles in your forearm. It is the same with your feet; when you move them, you move all the small muscles in the legs which aid circulation of the blood. With your feet encased in shoes, the foot muscles do not have full play.

Hardly a patient comes to me who does not complain of his feet and legs. If you want to cure varicose veins, you must help the blood get back to normal circulation again. You must have muscle tone and that comes when you exercise the feet. I am assuming that you are eating a well-balanced diet, so that your blood will be rich in body-building materials.

Here is a good foot exercise. Get a box of sand large enough to stand in, put a little cold water in it to make the sand cold and just stand in this and wiggle your feet for about ten minutes. This will not only help the muscle structure in the legs, but it will help the arches of the feet, as well.

If there is a swimming pool where you can wade up to your knees in cool water, then walk around on the hot cement and back into the cool water, alternating back and forth about twenty-five times, this will quicken the circulation by the contraction and relaxation produced. At home you can do this very nicely with hot and cool foot baths.

"Civilized" living forces us to do something to compensate for standing on our feet too long, sitting too long, getting too tired in every way. These abuses of the body hamper the natural flow of blood into the brain areas. Fatigue is a warning that tells us our circulation is impaired.

THE SLANTING BOARD IS ABSOLUTELY INDISPENSABLE for correcting and compensating for the punishments our daily living imposes upon us. Animation comes only when we have the proper blood flowing through the brain areas. We cannot be animated and energetic unless we counteract the downward pull of the blood. The brain cannot be properly fed if blood does not get to it. This is where the slanting board can do so much good.

In the brain we find an "interest center," and a

"fatigue center." When your brain does not have enough blood and is fatigued, you lose interest in doing things. This lack of blood supply to the brain area also causes our memory to fail us and renders us unable to make decisions. Lie full length on the slanting board, allowing gravity to assist in restoring the abdominal organs into their normal positions. For best results lie on the board at least one half hour.

WATER TREATMENTS. There are certain very effective water treatments which have been relegated to the background by modern machines and equipment. These treatments were worked out so we could use them in our homes with a minimum amount of service from others. The tendency in treatments today is to have someone else do everything for us.

Both hot and cold water are very good in keeping the blood moving and circulating. Cold water contracts the muscle structure and the arteries and this assists the blood in moving throughout the body. Heat relaxes and allows the blood to come back into the places that have been contracted.

If I had to recommend one type of bath only, it would be the sitz-bath. No one could go wrong by using this daily, as it is a tonic bath. This is a bath where you sit in cold water, every morning, or sometime during the day. There is no better bath for the prostate gland, menstrual disorders, ovarian troubles, constipation, and for developing tone in the abdominal organs. It is so important to take care of the abdominal organs. You should take the sitz-bath regularly for at least ten minutes and even up to as long as twenty minutes and it should be continued for months. The sitz-bath should always be taken with cold water as this acts as a tonic. Cold water is live water while hot water is dead water to be used only for relaxation.

Put about five inches of water in the bathtub and use an eight inch block or box to put your feet on. Do not put your feet in the water, nor your upper extremities; just the buttocks. You must exercise before and after you take the sitz-bath. This does not mean strenuous exercises; just a little moderate moving around before and after, so that you do not take the sitz-bath immediately upon arising or go to bed right after taking it. This moving around before and after the sitz-bath is to prevent the blood that has been drawn into the abdominal area, from being left there to become congested. The blood should be circulating well both before and after the bath is taken.

To sum up those tangible things which contribute to our physical well-being, we might add this commentary:

There are four chemical elements in which most people, I believe, are lacking: **calcium, silicon, sodium and iodine**. These seem to be the four most commonly lacking elements. In the East, 4000 people were tested for the amount of calcium in their bodies and it was found that there were only two who had enough calcium. Although calcium is one of the easiest elements to get into the body and is present in large quantities in the skeleton, etc., yet calcium which the tissues can use is the element most persons lack.

Bone meal is one of the best supplemental sources of **calcium**. There are many forms of bone meal on the market but I believe that Biost, put out by the Lee

Foundation in Milwaukee, Wisconsin, is the finest on the market today. Anything that is green contains a great deal of calcium as do grains, such as whole wheat, barley and buckwheat if these grains are cooked properly, in low-heat stainless steel (vapor sealed), the calcium will be kept intact.

Silicon is the magnetic element in the body, the element that is predominant in the sheath that surrounds the nerves. It helps to transport the energy from the brain to the different cell structures of the body. Messages from the brain to the muscles and organs of the body are not sent properly, or with the proper speed, when you do not have the proper supply of silicon. You are not alert; your body does not coordinate well; your muscle structure slows up and you are lazy and clumsy. The hair becomes dry and brittle, the skin becomes dry, and the fingernails split. The best way to get silicon is from Oat Straw tea. Drink this daily, with meals.

Iodine, another mineral element, is stored in the thyroid gland, but because of our "civilized" life, city noises, rushing about and working under tension, we often find the body deficient in iodine. Emotional strain depletes the thyroid's supply of iodine. We need very little iodine each day, and yet it is easy to become deficient in our supply. The blood in the body travels through the thyroid gland every hour and a half and it should have the material to deposit in the thyroid gland, so that this gland may have the chemicals to carry on its proper functions. Iodine is found abundantly in onions, pineapple juice, sea foods, sea kelp and Nova Scotia dulce. Sores on the body may develop from a lack of iodine, calcium, or other elements, and it is very difficult for even the skin specialist to detect the cause.

Sodium, the youth element, is the mineral that keeps the joints pliant, sweetens the stomach, and gets rid of the acids in the body. Sodium is found in abundance in okra and celery, two vegetables that are easy to get but are seasonal. It is also plentiful in whey.

Your body is a storehouse of magnesium, calcium, manganese, zinc, and trace elements. Unless you keep a supply of these minerals in your body you will suffer. We know that the calcium is stored in the bones and if you are using up more calcium than the body has, working longer hours than you should, expending a great deal of muscular effort, living a life of tension, keeping yourself constantly over-tired, you are wearing out the calcium in the body. When the calcium supply is depleted, it is taken away from the teeth, bones and tissues of your body; the tissues begin to lack tone and prolapses sets in. When your body is short of calcium, you have lost the healing and chemical in the body, and when you get a cut or sore, it does not heal well.

Vitamins B and E are the two very important vitamins for the body. Rice polishing is the best source of Vitamin B. Over a period of a year's time, by adding rice polishing to your diet, you can pick up the Vitamin B that you need. This is the most natural way of getting vitamin B into the body. Take one or two teaspoons of these polishing a day. Wheat germ, which also contains Vitamin B, is an excellent source of Vitamin E. This also can be secured through wheat germ oil. The wheat germ can be mixed with your food, such as cereals. I do not believe in taking large quantities of it as an excessive amount of wheat germ has been found to cause an irritation in the body.

Vitamin A is found in many of our natural, unrefined foods. Vitamins C and D are found in the colored fruits.

A diet of polished rice can wreck the health of a pigeon and bring illness to a human being.

The difference between what polished rice and natural brown rice can do to a pigeon! Within three hours after feeding vitamin B rich substance (rice polishing) the pigeon was able to stand and recovery seemed to be complete in twelve hours.

Diet's lacking needed chemical elements were fed to rats in an experiment and produced illness, malnutrition and near death.

In the same experiment, rats were fed with a well-balanced ration and became larger and healthier because of proper food.

CHEMICAL ELEMENT ANALYSIS

Essential Mineral Salts

<u>CALCIUM</u>: Found and needed mostly in the structural system. Tooth and bone mineral.

TONE-BUILDING IN THE BODY

Builds and maintains bone structure. Gives vitality, endurance. Heals wounds. Counteracts acid.

Principle Sources

Milk, Cheese, Raw egg yolk, Apricots, Figs, Prunes, Cranberries, Gooseberries, Cabbage, Spinach, Parsnips, Lettuce, Onions, Dates, Bran, Tops of Vegetables

<u>CHLORINE</u>: Found and needed mostly in digestive system. Secretions.

CLEANSER IN THE BODY

Cleans, expels waste, Freshens. Purifies. Disinfects.

Principle Sources

Goat Milk, Cow Milk, Salt Fish, Cheese, Cocoanut, Beets, Radishes, Common Salt.

<u>FLUORINE</u>: Found and needed mostly in the structural system. Tooth enamel. Preserves bones.

DISEASE REGISTER AND BEAUTIFIER IN BODY

Strengthens tendons. Knits bones.

Principle Sources

Cauliflower, Cabbage, Cheese, Raw Goat Milk, Raw Egg Yolk, Cod Liver, Oil, Brussels sprouts, Spinach, Tomatoes, Watercress.

<u>IODINE</u>: Found and needed mostly in nervous system. Gland and brain mineral.

METABOLISM NORMALIZER IN BODY.

Prevents goiter. Normalizes gland and cell action.

Ejects and counteracts poisons.

Principle Sources

Powdered Nova Scotia Dulce and Sea Lettuce (very high), Sea Foods, Carrots, Pears, Onions, Tomatoes, Pineapple,

Potato Skin, Cod Liver Oil. Garlic, Watercress.

MAGNESIUM: Found and needed mostly in the digestive system. Nerve mineral. Nature's laxative.

NEW CELL PROMOTER IN THE BODY.

Relaxes nerves. Refreshes system. Prevents and relieves constipation and auto-intoxication.

Principle Sources

Grapefruit, Oranges, Figs, Whole Barley, Corn, Wheat, Cocoanut, Goat's Milk, Raw Egg Yolk.

MANGANESE: Found and needed mostly in nervous system. Tissue strengthener. Memory mineral.

CONTROLLING NERVES IN THE BODY

Increases resistance. Co-ordinates thought and action. Improves memory.

Principle Sources

Nasturtium Leaves, Raw Egg Yolk. Almonds, Walnuts, Watercress. Mint, Parsley, Wintergreen, Endive, Pignolia nuts.

PHOSPHORUS: Found and needed mostly in nervous system. Brain and bone mineral.

BODY AND NERVE BUILDER

Nourishes brain and nerves. Builds power of thought. Stimulates growth of hair and bone.

Principle Sources

Sea Foods, Milk, Raw Egg Yolk, Parsnips, Whole Wheat, Barley, Yellow Corn, Nuts, Peas, Beans, Lentils.

POTASSIUM: Found and needed mostly in digestive system. Tissue and secretion mineral.

HEALER IN THE BODY

Liver Activator. Strongly alkaline. Makes tissues elastic, muscles supple. Creates grace, beauty, good disposition.

Principle Sources

Potato Skins, Dandelion, Dill, Sage, Cress, Dried Olives, Parsley, Blueberries, Peaches, Prunes, Cocoanut, Gooseberries, Cabbage, Figs, Almonds.

SILICON: Found and needed mostly in structural system. Nails, skin, teeth and hair.

SURGEON IN THE BODY

Gives keep hearing, sparkling eyes, hard teeth, glossy hair. Tones system and gives resistance to body.

Principle Sources

Oats, Barley, Spinach, Asparagus, Lettuce, Tomatoes, Cabbage, Figs, Strawberries.

SODIUM: Found and needed mostly in digestive system. Gland, ligament and blood builder.

YOUTH MAINTAINER

Aids digestion, Counteracts acidosis. Halts fermentation. Purifies the blood.

Principle Sources

Okra, Celery, Carrots, Beets, Cucumbers, String beans, Asparagus, Turnips, Strawberries, Oatmeal, Cheese, Raw Egg Yolk, Cocoanut, Black Figs.

SULPHUR: Found and needed mostly in the nervous system. Brain and tissue mineral.

PURIFIES AND ACTIVATES THE BODY

Purifies and tones the system. Intensifies feeling and emotion.

Principle Sources

Cabbage, Cauliflower, Onions, Asparagus, Carrots, Horse-radish, Shrimp. Chestnuts, Mustard Greens.

Harmonious and Balanced Living:

All of the foregoing has dealt with your physical well-being, but that is only one-third of the picture. The physical aspects may be compared to the canvas and the pigments and brushes used in painting a picture. It is necessary to use the mind to develop the techniques of an artist. You must have spiritual development, for this is what makes the difference between an inspired artist and one who is merely a dauber of paint.

As I said before, the time is coming when it is going to be shameful to be sick, and I know that day is coming, because doctors are failing. Too many doctors treat symptoms only and do not try to deal with the cause. I consider this maltreatment because if you do not get at the cause and treat that, but treat symptoms instead, you will find that after ridding yourself of one symptom, another will appear in its place. You may get rid of a headache by taking some kind of a depressant drug but if you do not find the cause of the headache and treat that, the headache will come again and again until you remove the cause. A head cold may be "treated," and apparently disappears from the head, only to be found in the bronchial tubes or the lungs, or possibly, the poison that tried to get out of the body through the nose, goes into the bloodstream and settles in the kidneys or in the liver. Because the head cold disappears, we think we are cured of whatever caused it, but this is not so, because this poison has merely gone to another part of the body, in its effort to eliminate itself from the body. There is only one way to get rid of toxic waste-acid and body poisons and that is by living the natural way and conforming to Nature's Laws. Then we will know the real joy of what it is to be healthy and live creative, progressive, happy lives.

I repeat that an attitude of mind produces a response in the body. If you have fear in your heart, you will talk with fear in your step. Your heart can become irregular by your thinking!

Learn to have a relaxed mind, to have a feeling of freedom within yourself; otherwise, you cannot have a body free from tension. You must learn to be a good giver and a good receiver. Learn how to be tactful. Learn that your mind is a powerful agent which can bring a world of peace and harmony or can build a world of irritation.

Most of the thoughts that come to us by way of radio and newspapers are not for the good of our health. They are irritating to both body and mind.

Learn to do things now. Stop putting off the things that will bring you health and peace of mind. They must be done each day. Your body is constantly going through a process of rebirth. You are throwing off the old and building the new. You build new skin in the palm of your hand every day; you can build a new heart but not in a day. It takes about seven months to build new organs and it will take a year for most people to really get to the place where they feel WONDERFUL.

A GOOD PHILOSOPHY

A person with a body as "healthy as a brute," but lacking in spirituality and peace of mind is no credit to a city, state or nation, for that body will not remain healthy and sooner or later it will break down. Considering a truly spiritual "life pattern," I believe many of us are far afield from the successful "life patterns," as laid down for us by the many Wise Ones of the different ages.

Most of us think we have to worry all the time. We are always expecting trouble, rather than good. If we think right and live right, the ALL Powerful One is bound to help us in our situations in life, and this attitude of right thinking and right living allows the body and mind to recuperate.

You must learn to recognize the good that is in yourself, the right that is there, the wonderful things that are there, or else you may turn out to be a weed instead of blossoming forth with the beauty of a rose. When you recognize and cultivate the good that is in yourself, you will be able to see it in others. You will then be able to "Love thine enemies." And the world needs honest, unselfish Love.

You must develop a PHILOSOPHY instead of aFILLOSOPHY. If you merely FILL your body and your mind and do not discriminate between false teachings and true teachings, good food and bad food, you cannot hope to build either a sound healthy body, or a good reasoning mind with which to develop a spiritual body.

The same laws apply in Spiritual teachings as in food therapy. Go back to the natural, the primary sources. You would not ask another man to chew and predigest your food for you, so why should you permit him to interpret the teachings of all the Wise Men of all the Ages?

Cults and creeds are nothing but the teachings of Avatars and great men, bleached, denuded and devitalized by the personal opinions of lesser men. Go to the original source teachings of these Avatars and do your own harvesting.

PHILO means LOVE in Greek. TO HAVE A TRUE AND WISE PHILOSOPHY is to LIVE BY THE LAW OF LOVE.

BE HONEST, BE KIND, avoid prejudices, BE FAITHFUL, BE DEPENDABLE, SEEK WISDOM AND INTELLIGENCE, AND PRESEVERE in these things and you cannot fail to make progress toward a BETTER FUTURE which means peace, happiness, and success. START NOW FOR THIS GOAL, and you are halfway along the road.

THE SEASONS ARE FOR MAN'S GOOD

To be able to "take it," and develop resistance in the body we have to get out into the air and sunshine. The seasonal elements are necessary to harden our bodies. However, there is a limit that the human body can stand and continue to stand.

Too much sunshine can be enervating; too much heat can be enervating; too much of the glare of the sunshine can drain a person of his nerve energy through a strain on his eyes. Where the body tissues are hardened and accustomed to a low altitude, the body is not able to adjust quickly in a high altitude when under the stress of unusual and excessive exercise.

It is well to get ready for a change of a coming season, whether it is winter, summer, spring or fall. Whichever season is just ahead of us, we should look out for our needs for that season. In the animal kingdom we can see how nature prepares the way for the birds and beasts as the different seasons approach and it is wonderful.

The coat of hair on a horse gets heavy just before cold weather sets in. One can predict the severity of the coming winter by the heaviness of the horse's hair as the fall season advances. As spring comes along, nature slowly and gradually thins the hair of these animals so that they may have perfect comfort for their body while working. Wise nature gradually prepares animals for seasonal changes, adjusting both their protective covering and their food needs.

When winter comes, the nuts are in season and the

more concentrated, building, heat foods, like the grains and nuts should be taken. These foods are not only for our pleasure and enjoyment but they mold our bodies and keep us in good health, when they are well chosen and eaten in the right proportions. Let us keep in mind that it is possible to kill ourselves by the amount of food that we eat. When we partake of dried fruits in the wintertime we find we have an extra amount of energy and we can well afford to do extra work and extra exercise.

It is in the winter that we have most of our heavy catarrhal conditions, and a good circulation of blood will help to carry this waste out of the body. It is necessary to keep the pores open. Extra perspiration in cold weather helps to keep our skin active and our kidneys clean, so we should take more exercise in winter than in the summertime.

Businessmen/women, who get very little physical exercise during the week, should go swimming about three times a week. As I have often said, swimming is very good exercise and will help to keep one in good physical condition.

As the spring season comes along, new foods are given to the animals and man should also have these seasonal foods for the growth and wellbeing of his body. Fruits and vegetables are waterier in the springtime and so we consider them more on the eliminative side. They are good for eliminating body acids and poisons. They will cause us to lose a little weight but in this way we will be ready to take on the hot summer weather with a different kind of blood than what we had during the winter.

In the summertime, during the extreme heat of the day, we should consider resting in the afternoon. We might take a lesson from the animals and start our work earlier in the morning. They do not work out in the sunshine in the middle of the day. One finds cattle, for example, grazing in the morning and late afternoon. Remembering that it is possible to kill ourselves by the amount of food we eat, it is well to consider eating lighter in hot weather.

"After Forty" Suggestions

It has been said that life begins at forty. It has been better said, that "age is a stage of tolerance." Truly, we should have enough experience in this era of light to readjust our lives mentally, so that we don't wear out our bodies, needlessly, as is done by "up and doing, daring, youth," through wasteful expenditure of energy that usually goes with young ideas.

The basal metabolism or the thyroid activity is a little slower after forty than before. The quickening activities of our tissues are usually not too responsive; they are not the same as when we were twenty. So it is well to consider doing our job under less mental strain. It is well to put in fewer hours on the job and enjoy ourselves.

While balance is something to consider at any time of our life, after forty it is more necessary. We have to learn to enjoy our enjoyment; to get all the value from a good fishing trip, and to know that a vacation is healing to anybody, providing it is a health vacation.

Pleasurable companions and good company are very important for recuperation. Our physical endeavors at the age of forty should never be overdone, because repair is slower and may result in damage that will be difficult to repair.

Let us consider our balance for the day in these *three* things: a useful *occupation*, needed *rest*, and enjoyable *recreation*. To balance our day through these three channels will result in a healthier, better balanced body that will surely serve us better in our work and play.

Relaxation and Tension Exercises

The cat is one of the quickest animals on its feet and "gets that way" from knowing how to relax. The boxer has the greatest strength and activity in his arms when he has learned how to relax. You can make your whole body as hard as steel through right exercise. You can stop pain in any part of the body by learning to tense the muscles for a few seconds around the congested area and then relax.

For cases of infantile paralysis, muscular atrophy, spasms, insomnia and similar troubles, there is no finer exercise than Tension-Relaxation. We know that most of the glands in the body are dependent upon a squeezing action to create circulation and for a release of the hormones within. We also know that the lymph glands in the body are dependent upon tension and motion for the release of the fluids which are the most important in the body. A stagnant blood and lymph system are not a healthy system.

We are now beginning to recognize the importance of lactic acid in the body. We definitely know that it neutralizes nerve acids. Lactic acid nerve injections are being used for the mentally ill. Those who are nervous, emotionally upset, and suffer from nerve depletion are the people who have not taken the right foods and have not had the proper kind and amount of exercise. Lactic acid is produced in the body as an end product of muscular metabolism. In importance it may be compared to the calcium in our food. It gives us the energy to accomplish physical expression. It helps to neutralize many of the fatigue acids in the body.

The ordinary callisthenic exercises are apt to create too many fatigue acids and so we recommend our own Relaxation and Tension Exercises, which produce the greatest amount of lactic acid and the least amount of fatigue acids.

Chinning—Exercise A

Tense the muscles by clawing the hands, holding them above the head and act as though you are chinning yourself. Tense all the muscles as you bring the hands down toward the shoulders. When you have reached the shoulders with this extreme muscle tension, then relax. It should take three or four seconds to bring the arms down. Do these three times.

Tension—Exercise B

The same exercise can be done with the arms directly out at the sides. Do not close the hands in fist fashion. Keep the fingers half closed so that you can tense the body more, if you desire. Bring the tensed arms in from the sides to the shoulders and when they reach the shoulders, drop them and relax them.

Tension—Relaxation Exercise C

Place the fingers of the right hand in the fingers of the left hand. Raise hands in front of you and a little to the left, and about even with the head. Pull down with the fingers of the right hand and resist with the left hand. Both hands should be tensed and should be pulling against each other. As you pull and resist, you are gradually bringing the left hand down with the right hand. Bring it down as far as you can and relax.

Do this same exercise by placing the hands in front of the body and to the right, at an angle. This time you pull the right hand down with the left hand, using resistance in the fingers of each hand. Bring down as far as possible and relax. This exercise should be repeated three times on each side.

Back Exercise D

Place both arms straight down in back of you. Tense the muscles and pull one arm against the other. Then raise the hands up toward the shoulders, all the while keeping your hands locked and tensed. Then slowly bring them down to position and relax. This can be done under tension, three or four times and then rest.

Leg Exercise E

Put one leg forward in a relaxed position, then tense the muscles of this leg and relax. Repeat this exercise for the other leg. This exercise may be repeated from three to six times for each leg.

Master Exercise

Lie on the floor or a bed, arms down at the sides and legs and feet straight, not bent. Bending at the hips, bring the head and feet up toward the ceiling, tensing all the muscles of the body, including the arms, legs, stomach, etc. Hold for three seconds in this position and relax. Do these three times. How do you spend your time? Some people kill time. Others just let it die a slow death. Ever hear the song (usually by some operatic hopeful) "I Love Life, I Want to Live"? Dr. Frank Gallup polled 29,000 Americans who were 94 years old and older and concluded that the way to have a long life is:

To be a woman

To be born in Norway

Of long-lived ancestors

Not to worry

Not to smoke

Eat wisely and lightly

Have enthusiasm

Have a real religious belief

Sounds good; but how much time do you have left to live? A prominent business concern computed: Subtract your present age from 80. Take what you have and multiply it by 7. Divide the answer by 10. Of course you can forget the whole thing if you're a careless driver! It's later than you think.

The clock of life is wound but once,

And no man has the power

To tell just when the hands will stop

At late or early hour.

Now is the only time you own;

Live, love, toil with a will.

Place not your faith in tomorrow

The clock may then be still.

Author Unknown

THE PRAYER OF AN INDIAN

O Great Spirit, whose voice I hear in the winds and whose breath gives your life to all the world, hear me. I come before you, one of your many children I am small and weak, I need your strength and wisdom.

Let me walk in beauty and make my eyes ever behold the red and purple sunset. Make my hand respect the things you have made, my ears sharp to hear your voice. Make me wise, so that I may know the things you have taught my people, the lesson you have hidden in every leaf and rock.

I seek strength not to be superior to my brothers, but to be able to fight my greatest enemy....myself. Make me ever ready to come to you with clean hands and straight eyes, so when life fades as a fading sunset, my spirit may come to you without shame.

By Chief Yellow Lark

From the Study of Bernard Jensen, D. C.

IMPOSITIONS FOR GETTING WELL

Learn to accept whatever decision is made. Let the other person make a mistake and learn. Learn to forget and forgive. Be thankful and bless people. Live in harmony - even if it is good for you. Do not talk about your sickness. Gossip will kill you. Don't let anybody else gossip to you either. Gossip that comes through the grape vine is usually sour. Be by yourself every day for ten minutes with the thought of how to make yourself a better person. Replace negative thoughts with uplifting, positive thoughts. Skin brush daily. Use a slant board daily. Have citrus fruit in sections only - never in juice form. Have only a limited amount of bread (with a lot of bowel trouble, no bread). Exercise daily. Keep your spine limber. Develop abdominal muscles. Do sniff breathing. Have a daily set of exercises. Grass walk and sand walk for happy feet. No smoking, drinking, spitting or cussing. Keep away from "spitty" people. Bed at sundown - 9 o'clock at the latest. Sleep outdoors, out of the city in circulating air. Work out your problems in the morning - don't take them to bed with you.

FOR RANCH GUESTS:

Who is your doctor? Someone is always giving advice - the plumber, musician, reflexologist, vitamin salesman, visitors and who have you. If you want their advice and mine, bring all parties concerned to me and let's talk it over. If you want to follow someone else's advice, it's all right with me. I would like to be dismissed if you're mixing too many ideas with mine.

FOOD HEALING LAWS

1. Natural food. 60% of food eaten must be raw.

2. Your diet should be 80% alkaline and 20% acid. Look to acid-alkaline chart in "Vital Foods For Total Health," page 100.

3. Proportion - 6 vegetables daily; 2 fruits daily; 1 starch daily and 1 protein daily.

4. Variety - vary sugars, proteins, starches, vegetables and fruits from meal to meal and from day to day.

5. Overeating - you can kill yourself with the amount of food you eat.

6. Combinations - separate starches and proteins. Eat one at lunch and the other at supper. Have fruits for breakfast and at 3:00 o'clock.

7. Cook without water. Cook without high heat. Cook without air touching hot food.

RULES OF EATING

1. If not entirely comfortable in mind and body from the previous mealtime, you should miss the next meal.

2. Do not eat unless you have a keen desire for the plainest food.

3. Do not eat beyond your needs.

4. Be sure to thoroughly masticate your food.

5. Miss meals if in pain - emotionally upset - not hungry - chilled - overheated - and during acute illness.

OTHER BOOKLETS BY DR. JENSEN

1. HOW TO ENJOY BETTER HEALTH NATURAL REMEDIES

2. HOW TO RELAX AND RELIEVE TENSION

3. HOW TO REVITALIZE YOUR GLANDS

4. A NEW SLANT ON HEALTH AND BEAUTY—SLANT BOARD

5. A HEALTH PATTERN TO LIVE BY

6. HOW TO BUILD A BETTER BODY FROM YOUR KITCHEN

7. HOW THE BREATH OF LIVE SUSTAINS YOU

8. PHYSICAL, MENTAL AND SPIRITUAL BALANCE

9. DEVELOPING INWARD CALM

10. THE NEED FOR A NEW ATTITUDE

11. THE HEART OF CIRCULATORY SYSTEM

12. THREE STEPS TO THE HIGHER LIFE (Part I)

13. THREE STEPS TO THE HIGHER LIFE (Part II)

14. THREE STEPS TO THE HIGHER LIFE (Part III)

15. HEALTH FOR OUR CHILDREN

16. SPECIAL FOODS FOR SPECIAL NEEDS

17. LETS BEGIN AT THE BEGINNING

18. YOUR LOVE LIFE

19. INTESTINAL DISORDERS FASTING/ELIMINATIVE DIETS

20. VOLUME I — SECRETS I CAN SHARE WITH YOU

21. VOLUME II — MORE SECRETS I CAN SHARE WITH YOU

Meet the Author

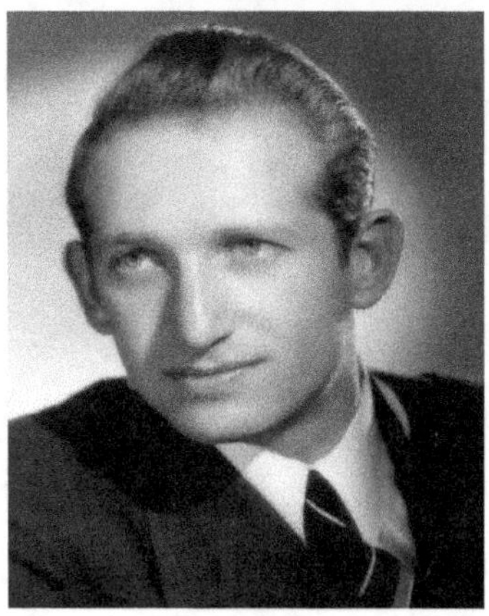

Bernard Jensen, Ph.D., D.C, N.D., Nutritionist of Los Angeles, Calif. Born in Stockton, Calif, in 1908.

Possessing a convincing philosophy that would credit much older practitioners, Bernard Jensen, D.C, Lecturer and Teacher of Right Living, acquired from the beginning of his studies the vision "that Nature does all the healing." He believes doctors can only work with natural laws. His work is sane, up-to-date and practical teaches a balanced "how-to-live" regime.

At only 18, Dr. Jensen began studies with the West Coast Chiropractic College, Oakland, Calif. At 21 he began his practice of chiropractic in that city and has been practicing that science ever since. Widely traveled, he has been honored with post-graduate degrees from the National College in Chicago and the American School of Naturopathy, New York. He studied methods of the Battle Creek Sanitarium, of Tilden's School of Fasting in Denver. At an early age he was teaching his "How-to-live" methods to professional groups.

For 50 years. Dr. Jensen has led a most strenuous life, lecturing, radio broadcasting and directing his own health center in Escondido, California.

His current plans include Radio and TV guest appearances, a nationwide tour, and more contributions to Iridology and color, with new works planned in both areas. Dr. Jensen's The Science and Practice of Iridology has brought him international acclaim and is currently being translated into Spanish. Nine more books are in various stages of production, including his spiritual masterpiece. Arise and Shine, and color book.

About the Author

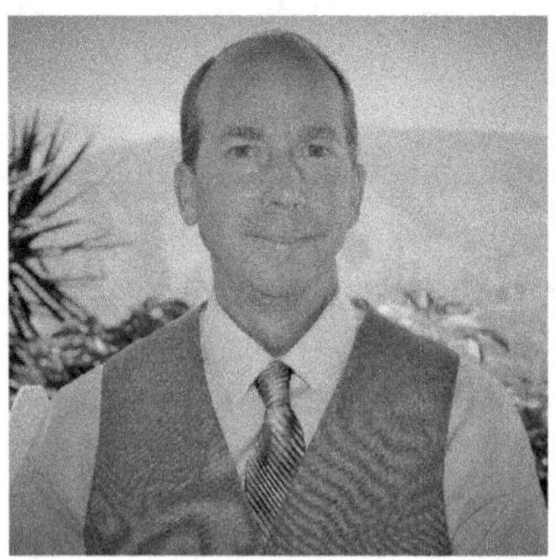

Jon Jensen, CMH, has been involved in holistic health for over 30 years with experience in Iridology, nutrition, and personal self-development. Jon started taking classes in Iridology and nutrition from his grandfather, the late Dr. Bernard Jensen, in 1980. Dr. Bernard Jensen is generally regarded throughout North America as the forefather of Iridology. Jon filled numerous roles over the years and participated in his grandfather's many classes and projects. Jon was involved in research for his grandfather's books, helping to pioneer a new way of iris analysis using the computer, and assisting with seminars.

Jon's mission is to educate people on the basic tenants of health and nutrition that his grandfather taught throughout his lifetime as a holistic health practitioner. Basics like the importance of a plant-based diet, regular exercise, proper sleep/rest, taking care of the bowel and more. Throughout his travels he searched for the longest living humans and wanted to know why they lived so long.

In 1995 Jon stayed by his grandfather's side after Dr. Bernard Jensen became paralyzed from the waist down from a car accident. Jon was right there every day of his grandfather's plan to walk again. With a big sign on the wall in front of Dr. Jensen's bed where he could see it every day that said, "LUCKY BOY". Every day consisted of many different healing modalities and supplements. Jon would travel to the Hidden Valley Health Ranch in the early morning and watch while Apolinar, Dr. Jensen's main ranch worker, milked the goat for Dr. Jensen's fresh morning goat milk drink. Jon would drive his grandfather and grandmother Marie to Los Angeles twice a week for chiropractic adjustments and frequency therapy, treating the whole body, mind, and spirit, and being involved in every aspect of what the doctors called a **"Miracle"—as his grandfather walked again on his own.** Jon is writing more on the entire recovery process and will publish it through Amazon.

After his grandfather's recovery, Jon shifted his attention to additional training by taking classes with some of the prominent leaders in the fields of Sclerology with Dr. Leonard Mehlmauer, Rayid (emotional iridology) with Denny Johnson, European based integrated iridology with Dr. Ellen Tart-Jensen as well as animal iridology with Dr. Mercedes Colburn. Jon attended Kalos© classes with Dr. Valerie Seeman-Gersch learning about Transformational Healing methods.

Jon was President of the Escondido Chapter of Chamber Toastmasters and enjoys speaking to groups.

Jon wrote an article for The Price-Pottenger Nutrition Foundation Journal on Animal Iridology and Nutrition. Jon has given presentations at: Holistic Health Fairs, Expo's, Herb Shops, Churches and Health Food Stores.

Jon is currently Executive Director at the "Live Pure Kids" foundation in Arizona. Jon works closely with Gavin Tucker the President/Founder, and Jackie Morales, Vice President.

The Live Pure Kids Foundation

<u>Mission Statement</u>: To change the world for our next generation starting from within.

<u>Vision Statement</u>: With the support of parents, families and the community, educating all kids through an organic plant-based mindfulness yoga lifestyle, we are giving our next generation the tools of today to be the world leaders of tomorrow.

www.livepurekids.com

Jon recently published a nutrition book called, "A Simple Guide to Healthy Living" along with the 21 Dr. Jensen Booklet series and they are available for purchase on Amazon.

For more information Jon can be found at www.jensenholistichealth.com   www.bernardjensen.org

www.ingramcontent.com/pod-product-compliance
Lightning Source LLC
Chambersburg PA
CBHW050657250726
48662CB00002B/732